Table of Contents

INTRODUCTION

Having a gut feeling, shouldn't just be an emotional response.

So, if the gut isn't working efficiently, we're not getting the necessary nutrients to our cells. Research shows that gut health, has a significant impact on mood, energy levels, and immunity. Dr. B's book, Fiber Fueled, shows us that fiber is the basis of good health, and he gives us practical and, yes, "easy-to-digest," science on the gut. Fiber Fueled explains why fiber matters, and how best to incorporate fiber fuelled plants, and fermented foods into our diets.

Dr. B is a renowned gastroenterologist, and through years of research and experience, he maintains that optimal health relies on a healthy gut. And, the solution that he offers is simple; eat more fiber.

In brief, as you know, it's often difficult to start these processes and to adopt a shift in lifestyle. That's why Dr. B lays out a 28-day kick-start program that helps us benefit from a diverse plant-based diet, that's high in fiber and will restore and maintain a healthy gut.

What Are Microbes and How Do They Impact on Gut Health?

How many of these little engine-drivers, or microbes, do you think that you have in your digestive system? Dr. B says that there are an astonishing thirty-nine trillion micro-organisms that take up residence in our colons. It's difficult to conceptualize a number this enormous. So, imagine looking up at a clear night sky, and seeing every star in the Milky Way. Then take the number of stars you can see, and multiply this by a hundred - that's roughly how many micro-organisms live in your colon.

What's even more mind-blowing is that the number of microbes far exceeds the number of cells in the human body. So, if you think about it, we're 90% bacteria, and only 10% human.

The thought of bacteria often triggers negativity. But, the truth is that bacteria are often what makes us the most healthy. When in balance, the bacteria in our bodies have incredible healing power. They help digestion, and strengthen our immune system. On the other hand, when your gut biome is unbalanced, this can cause weight gain, and increased blood sugar and cholesterol levels.

What Causes Gut Imbalance?

When it comes to gut imbalance, there are two main culprits; medication and poor diet.

Did you know that three out of five Americans take prescription drugs? The problem is that these medications often wreak havoc on gut microbes. Medication frequently wipes them out, even the good ones. After a single course of antibiotics, our gut takes approximately four weeks to return to its pretreatment state. And most antibiotics only treat symptoms and not the underlying causes of the illness. Dr. B says that we're a hyper-medicated civilization that relies on a system that focuses on sick-care, not healthcare.

The second culprit is our increasingly poor diets. Dr. B says that the way we eat, can be harmful to our gut and overall health. Many of us could be in a situation where we may eat enough, but our healthy microbes could be starving. According to the U.S. Department of Agriculture, approximately 32% of our calorie intake comes from animal foods, 57% from processed plant foods, and only 11% from whole grains, fruits, vegetables, and nuts.

Diets that are high in animal protein and processed foods, tend to feed the inflammatory-producing bacteria, while starving the good, health-promoting bacteria. Furthermore, high animal protein intake is associated with an increase in inflammatory microbes. Studies show that L-carnitine, found in red meat, egg yolk, and dairy products, causes gut bacteria that can increase the risk of Alzheimer's, strokes, and heart disease.

We should all know that processed foods such as white bread, rice, pasta, and sugar-laden cereals, are highly refined and low in fiber. One of the significant problems with this is that they're rapidly absorbed into the small intestine, instead of being slowly digested. This quick absorption reduces our gut microbial diversity. Inflammatory bacteria thrive on the sugar that's produced from simple carbohydrates.

What's encouraging is that plant protein, fuels anti-inflammatory microbes and suppresses the destructive microbes. This bonus helps us to ward off many diseases. The need to nourish our healthy gut microbes is paramount.

And here's the thing, you've probably heard of probiotics, but have you heard anything about prebiotics?

Signs of Poor Gut Health

There are many side effects of having poor gut health. A relatively common condition is "leaky gut". This is a condition where small pieces of food penetrate the intestinal wall, and enter the bloodstream. They certainly don't belong there. This infiltration triggers a cascade of events - all of which are bad news for us.

When food particles and other substances are absorbed incorrectly, our immune systems go into high alert, and attack them as pathogens. This immune response, creates inflammation in the bloodstream, that then moves through the body. It causes digestive distress such as bloating, heartburn, and diarrhea. Interestingly, the most common area for poor gut health symptoms involve the brain. Insomnia, brain fog, or poor memory can be signs of a poorly functioning digestive system.

Many of us may try very hard to be healthy, and opt for healthier options for what we eat. However, if the gut isn't happy, essential nutrients can't get to our cells, and we continue to feel tired and unwell.

The good news is that medical health breakthroughs are continuously providing us with new information to help restore and optimize gut function. When it comes to learning about our digestive health, and the little creatures living in our guts known as microbes, knowledge is expanding.

What are Probiotics and Prebiotics?

Probiotics are our healthy gut bacteria, and prebiotics are the foods that enable them to thrive. Here is where Dr. B's favorite F-word comes in. The F-word is Fiber. Fiber is a prebiotic, and it's absolutely essential.

There's a lot of misconception around fiber and high-fiber diets. For many of us, when we think about fibre, we think of foods that resemble cardboard and cereals that are difficult to swallow. Many of us might remember women in advertising, rubbing their stomachs, advocating for a miracle product bound to keep us all "regular." But, fiber does so much more than just passing through us, and cleaning out our systems.

The role of fiber in gut health is diverse, and we shouldn't neglect it. Unsurprisingly, plants have a total monopoly on this nutrient. Fiber is part of a plant's cellular structure. If you want to get fiber naturally, the only way to do it, is via plants.

What's also important is realizing the difference between soluble and insoluble fiber. Insoluble fiber is the roughage that passes through our mouths, down to the gut. Along the way, insoluble fiber cleans things up and finally comes out the other end. Soluble fiber is different, and from a nutritional standpoint, it's a complex carbohydrate. Complex carbohydrates remain unchanged as they pass from our mouths to our stomachs, and even down the fifteen to twenty feet of your small intestine.

By the time soluble fiber reaches our colons, it still has the same molecular structure as when it went into our mouths. So, once in the colon, the healthy bacteria metabolize the fiber. This stage is when the magic happens.

What are Short-Chain Fatty Acids and Why Do We Need Them?

The breakdown of fiber by gut bacteria unleashes what Dr. B regards as the most healing nutrient in nature: short-chain fatty acids. Dr. B can't say enough good things about the magic of fatty acids, and he admits his interest in them often borders on obsession. Science now shows that short-chain fatty acids are the dominant drivers of gut health, and benefit the entire body.

The name describes them well. They're short-chain, chemical compounds made up of two, three, or four carbon atoms connected in different variations. This description may sound a bit complicated, but they're the dominant energy source for our colon.

They also help healthy microbes grow, they repair the leaky gut, and they're vital regarding reducing the release of bad bacteria and harmful toxins into our systems. In short, they're the superheroes that ease gut dysbiosis. They reduce gas, bloating, and irritable bowel syndrome. Furthermore, they help regulate the immune system, prevent cancer, heart disease, strokes, and Type 2 diabetes.

But, as with all things there's a bit of a catch. To get the benefits of short-chain fatty acids, we need to eat more prebiotics, and thus more fiber. To do that, we need to ramp up our plant consumption.

Ramping up our plant consumption may be met with a bit of an eye-roll. Mainly at the thought of eating countless kale leaves. The key to this approach is realizing the importance of variety, and having an open mind about plants. One of the most extensive studies on microbes, published by Dr. Knight in 2017, shows that the single most significant predictor of a healthy gut microbiome, is incorporating a diverse range of plants into our diets.

Research suggests that we should be eating up to thirty different plants per week, to support a healthy microbiome. The good news is that every plant type we introduce into our diet, provides a unique microbe community, that helps our gut thrive. So the more varied our plant intake is, the more diverse our microbiomes become.

Our food worlds can open up significantly, if we learn to appreciate and explore the wide variety of plant ingredients available. Dr. B says that, there are over three hundred thousand edible plants on the planet. However, most Americans don't eat more than twenty-five. Think about what you could be missing out on? The key idea is that plant diversity in our menu, should be part of our planning every time we eat, and this is where Dr. B's diet plan comes in. He provides comprehensive information, along with a four-week diet plan to get us all fiber fueled.

Let's explore his strategy.

How To Begin Your Journey to Good Gut Health

An easy way to incorporate plants into our diets is to remember the acronym, F-GOALS. This acronym stands for fruits and fermented foods, greens and grains, omega-rich nuts and seeds, aromatics, legumes, and sulforaphane.

Fruit and Fermented Foods

Remember that adage about apples and doctors? Well, Dr. B, recommends more than just a single apple a day.

A study from Cornell University shows that eating combinations of fruit, results in increased antioxidant activity in the body.

Berries are incredibly nutrient-rich, and one study shows that eating two servings of berries per week, can reduce Parkinson's disease by 23%.

And as with most things, don't take shortcuts. All of those juice fads you read about, will never match the benefits of eating the whole fruit. For example, one orange contains 45 calories, 2.5 grams of fiber, and 9 grams of sugar. Orange juice, on the other hand, contains 134 calories, 0.5 grams of fiber, and 23.3 grams of sugar. So orange juice contains more than double the calories and sugar of a whole orange, without the fiber.

You may have noticed, there's been a massive resurgence in the popularity of fermented foods. This is one fad that should become a lifestyle. Fermented foods are rich in healthy bacteria, or probiotics. Almost every culture on earth, has fermented foods as part of their food tradition because it's an excellent preservation method.

This abundance of options is good news when you're looking for fermented foods in your local grocery store. Be adventurous with experimenting with these ingredients.

Dr. B's suggestion for an afternoon energy boost is to replace coffee with a cup of miso. Miso is a fermented soybean paste with a salty flavor. It's packed with calcium to promote healthy bones and can ward off cancer.

Greens and Grains

We all know that greens are excellent for our health; Popeye and the Jolly Green Giant have been touting their benefits for years. The trouble with greens, is that they can have a bad reputation with regards to taste. This reputation may have a lot to do with us generally eating over boiled greens.

There's so much diversity when it comes to eating, and preparing, our daily greens. Even the leaves of some root veggies like beetroot, turnip, radish, and carrots are edible. Popeye was right about spinach. Eating one cup of spinach offers 36% of our daily iron intake, 11% of our daily protein, 4 grams of fiber, and a host of vitamins and minerals.

When it comes to grains, it's pretty intuitive. Drop the refined stuff, such as white rice and highly processed bread, but don't be carb-phobic. Dr. B says that if you want a healthy gut, whole grains are essential.

To back this up, Dr. B provides numerous studies. One particular ten-year study of dietary patterns examined 37 different food groups and showed that whole grain consumption had the most potent anti-inflammatory effect on the body. Those consuming whole grains saw their inflammation measure, the C-reactive protein, drop by 21%. Those who eliminated whole grains saw theirs increase by 12%. The evidence is clear; whole grains are anti-inflammatory, so it's time to end the war on carbs and enjoy that slice of freshly baked sourdough.

Omega-3

The most efficient way to get more Omega-3 is by incorporating more seeds into your diet. Dr. B suggests adding flaxseed, chia seeds, and hemp seeds to your daily diet. The great thing about seeds is that they're easy to incorporate into salad dressings, porridge, or just as a sprinkling to add texture.

Aromatics

Foods such as onions, leeks, and garlic do more than ward off vampires. Aromatics such as these contain an enzyme called allianase, which is anti-viral, anti-fungal, and anti-parasitic. But, to activate this enzyme, we need to pause after chopping these vegetables. Dr. B calls this the "Chop and Stop" method. Chop up your garlic or onion, then wait 10 minutes before adding it to the frying pan.

Legumes

Legumes are packed with fiber. Even your typical green peas are full of fiber; a cup of pea's has 7 grams of fiber. Lentils contain a whopping 16 grams, so why not combine various legumes with a whole grain like brown rice? In this way, you can create a complete protein.

Sulforaphane

It sounds like a bit of a mouthful, but studies show that this compound creates healthy microbes and restores harmony to the gut. But, what's sulforaphane, and where can you find it? Sulforaphane is unique to the cruciferous family of vegetables, such as broccoli, Brussel sprouts, and cabbage.

Dietary fiber: Essential for a healthy diet

Eat more fiber. You've probably heard it before. But do you know why fiber is so good for your health?

Dietary fiber — found mainly in fruits, vegetables, whole grains and legumes — is probably best known for its ability to prevent or relieve constipation. But foods containing fiber can provide other health benefits as well, such as helping to maintain a healthy weight and lowering your risk of diabetes, heart disease and some types of cancer.

Selecting tasty foods that provide fiber isn't difficult. Find out how much dietary fiber you need, the foods that contain it, and how to add them to meals and snacks.

What is dietary fiber?

Dietary fiber, also known as roughage or bulk, includes the parts of plant foods your body can't digest or absorb. Unlike other food components, such as fats, proteins or carbohydrates — which your body breaks down and absorbs — fiber isn't digested by your body. Instead, it passes relatively intact through your stomach, small intestine and colon and out of your body.

Fiber is commonly classified as soluble, which dissolves in water, or insoluble, which doesn't dissolve.

• **Soluble fiber.** This type of fiber dissolves in water to form a gel-like material. It can help lower blood cholesterol and glucose levels. Soluble fiber is found in oats, peas, beans, apples, citrus fruits, carrots, barley and psyllium.

- **Insoluble fiber.** This type of fiber promotes the movement of material through your digestive system and increases stool bulk, so it can be of benefit to those who struggle with constipation or irregular stools. Whole-wheat flour, wheat bran, nuts, beans and vegetables, such as cauliflower, green beans and potatoes, are good sources of insoluble fiber.

The amount of soluble and insoluble fiber varies in different plant foods. To receive the greatest health benefit, eat a wide variety of high-fiber foods.

Benefits of a high-fiber diet

A high-fiber diet:

- Normalizes bowel movements. Dietary fiber increases the weight and size of your stool and softens it. A bulky stool is easier to pass, decreasing your chance of constipation. If you have loose, watery stools, fiber may help to solidify the stool because it absorbs water and adds bulk to stool.

• Helps maintain bowel health. A high-fiber diet may lower your risk of developing hemorrhoids and small pouches in your colon (diverticular disease). Studies have also found that a high-fiber diet likely lowers the risk of colorectal cancer. Some fiber is fermented in the colon. Researchers are looking at how this may play a role in preventing diseases of the colon.

• Lowers cholesterol levels. Soluble fiber found in beans, oats, flaxseed and oat bran may help lower total blood cholesterol levels by lowering low-density lipoprotein, or "bad," cholesterol levels. Studies also have shown that high-fiber foods may have other heart-health benefits, such as reducing blood pressure and inflammation.

• Helps control blood sugar levels. In people with diabetes, fiber — particularly soluble fiber — can slow the absorption of sugar and help improve blood sugar levels. A healthy diet that includes insoluble fiber may also reduce the risk of developing type 2 diabetes.

• Aids in achieving healthy weight. High-fiber foods tend to be more filling than low-fiber foods, so you're likely to eat less and stay satisfied longer. And high-fiber foods tend to take longer to eat and to be less "energy dense," which means they have fewer calories for the same volume of food.

• Helps you live longer. Studies suggest that increasing your dietary fiber intake — especially cereal fiber — is associated with a reduced risk of dying from cardiovascular disease and all cancers.

How much fiber do you need?

The Institute of Medicine, which provides science-based advice on matters of medicine and health, gives the following daily fiber recommendations for adults:

Fiber: Daily recommendations for adults

 Age 50 or younger Age 51 or older

Institute of Medicine

Men 38 grams 30 grams

Women 25 grams 21 grams

Your best fiber choices

If you aren't getting enough fiber each day, you may need to boost your intake. Good choices include:

• Whole-grain products

• Fruits

• Vegetables

• Beans, peas and other legumes

• Nuts and seeds

Refined or processed foods — such as canned fruits and vegetables, pulp-free juices, white breads and pastas, and non-whole-grain cereals — are lower in fiber. The grain-refining process removes the outer coat (bran) from the grain, which lowers its fiber content. Enriched foods have some of the B vitamins and iron added back after processing, but not the fiber.

Fiber supplements and fortified foods

Whole foods rather than fiber supplements are generally better. Fiber supplements — such as Metamucil, Citrucel and FiberCon — don't provide the variety of fibers, vitamins, minerals and other beneficial nutrients that foods do.

Another way to get more fiber is to eat foods, such as cereal, granola bars, yogurt and ice cream, with fiber added. The added fiber usually is labeled as "inulin" or "chicory root." Some people complain of gassiness after eating foods with added fiber.

However, some people may still need a fiber supplement if dietary changes aren't sufficient or if they have certain medical conditions, such as constipation, diarrhea or irritable bowel syndrome. Check with your doctor before taking fiber supplements.

Tips for fitting in more fiber

Need ideas for adding more fiber to your meals and snacks? Try these suggestions:

- **Jump-start your day.** For breakfast choose a high-fiber breakfast cereal — 5 or more grams of fiber a serving. Opt for cereals with "whole grain," "bran" or "fiber" in the name. Or add a few tablespoons of unprocessed wheat bran to your favorite cereal.

- **Switch to whole grains.** Consume at least half of all grains as whole grains. Look for breads that list whole wheat, whole-wheat flour or another whole grain as the first ingredient on the label and have at least 2 grams of dietary fiber a serving. Experiment with brown rice, wild rice, barley, whole-wheat pasta and bulgur wheat.

- **Bulk up baked goods.** Substitute whole-grain flour for half or all of the white flour when baking. Try adding crushed bran cereal, unprocessed wheat bran or uncooked oatmeal to muffins, cakes and cookies.

- **Lean on legumes.** Beans, peas and lentils are excellent sources of fiber. Add kidney beans to canned soup or a green salad. Or make nachos with refried black beans, lots of fresh veggies, whole-wheat tortilla chips and salsa.

• **Eat more fruit and vegetables.** Fruits and vegetables are rich in fiber, as well as vitamins and minerals. Try to eat five or more servings daily.

• **Make snacks count.** Fresh fruits, raw vegetables, low-fat popcorn and whole-grain crackers are all good choices. A handful of nuts or dried fruits also is a healthy, high-fiber snack — although be aware that nuts and dried fruits are high in calories.

High-fiber foods are good for your health. But adding too much fiber too quickly can promote intestinal gas, abdominal bloating and cramping. Increase fiber in your diet gradually over a few weeks. This allows the natural bacteria in your digestive system to adjust to the change.

Also, drink plenty of water. Fiber works best when it absorbs water, making your stool soft and bulky.

Increasing Fiber Intake

Why is fiber important?

A high-fiber diet appears to reduce the risk of developing various conditions, including heart disease, diabetes, diverticular disease, constipation and colon cancer. Fiber is important for the health of the digestive system and for lowering cholesterol.

What is fiber?

Dietary fiber is material from plant cells that cannot be broken down by enzymes in the human digestive tract. There are two important types of fiber: water-soluble and water insoluble. Each has different properties and characteristics.

• Soluble Water-soluble fibers absorb water during digestion. They increase stool bulk and may decrease blood cholesterol levels. Soluble fiber can be found in fruits (such as apples, oranges and grapefruit), vegetables, legumes (such as dry beans, lentils and peas), barley, oats and oat bran.

• Insoluble Water-insoluble fibers remain unchanged during digestion. They promote normal movement of intestinal contents. Insoluble fiber can be found in fruits with edible peel or seeds, vegetables, whole grain products (such as whole-wheat bread, pasta and crackers), bulgur wheat, stone ground corn meal, cereals, bran, rolled oats, buckwheat and brown rice.

How much fiber do I need each day?

The American Heart Association Eating Plan suggests eating a variety of food fiber sources. Total dietary fiber intake should be 25 to 30 grams a day from food, not supplements. Currently, dietary fiber intakes among adults in the United States average about 15 grams a day. That's about half the recommended amount.

How do I increase my fiber intake?

Here are some easy ways to increase fiber:

Grains and Cereals

• As a general rule, include at least one serving of whole grain in every meal.

• Keep a jar of oat bran or wheat germ handy. Sprinkle over salad, soup, breakfast cereals and yogurt.

• Use whole-wheat flour when possible in your cooking and baking.

• Choose whole grain bread. Look on the label for breads with the highest amount of fiber per slice.

• Choose cereals with at least 5 grams of fiber per serving.

• Keep whole-wheat crackers on hand for an easy snack.

• Cook with brown rice instead of white rice. If the switch is hard to make, start by mixing them together.

Legumes and Beans

• Add kidney beans, garbanzos or other bean varieties to your salads. Each 1/2 cup serving is approximately 7 to 8 grams of fiber.

• Substitute legumes for meat two to three times per week in chili and soups

• Experiment with international dishes (such as Indian or Middle Eastern) that use whole grains and legumes as part of the main meal or in salads.

Fruits and Vegetables

• Eat at least five servings of fruits and vegetables each day. Fresh fruit is slightly higher in fiber than canned. Eat the peel whenever possible — it's easier than peeling or eating around it.

• Have fresh fruit for dessert.

• Eat whole fruits instead of drinking juices. Juices don't have fiber.

• Add chopped dried fruits to your cookies, muffins, pancakes or breads before baking.

Dried fruits have a higher amount of fiber than the fresh versions. For example, 1 cup of grapes has 1 gram of fiber, but 1 cup of raisins has 7 grams. However, 1 cup of raisins or any other dried fruit has more calories than the fresh fruit variety.

• Add sliced banana, peach or other fruit to your cereal.

• Grate carrots on salads.

How much fiber do I get from fruits and vegetables?

While all fruits have some fiber, there are some that are higher than others. Here are a few that have 3 to 4 grams of fiber:

• Apple

• Orange

• Tangerine

• Pear

• 1 cup blueberries

- 1 cup strawberries

Raspberries are high in fiber, as one cup has 8 grams.

Here are some vegetable choices that have 3 to 4 grams of fiber:

- 1/2 cup peas

- 1/2 cup cauliflower

- 1 cup carrots

- 1 medium sweet potato

- 1/2 cup squash

Why is soluble fiber so important?

Soluble fiber has been shown to reduce total blood cholesterol levels and may improve blood sugar levels in people with diabetes.

The best sources of soluble fiber are oats, dried beans and some fruits and vegetables. Although there is no dietary reference intake for insoluble or soluble fiber, many experts recommend a total dietary fiber intake of 25 to 30 grams per day with about one-fourth — 6 to 8 grams per day — coming from soluble fiber.

For a Longer Life and Happier Gut, Eat More Fiber

Get fierce with fiber

It's easy to get caught up in counting calories and grams of added sugars, fats, proteins, and carbs when you're trying to eat well. But there's one nutrient that too often gets thrown to the wayside: dietary fiber.

Scientist's have long known that eating fiber is good for health. Decades ago, Irish physician (and fiber enthusiast) Denis Burkitt proclaimed, "America is a constipated nation... if you pass small stools, you have to have large hospitals." And yet, years later, many of us are still ignoring our fiber intake.

American adults are only eating an average of 15 grams of fiber on any given day, despite the daily recommendations from the Academy of Nutrition and Dietetics being:

• 25 grams for women, or 21 grams if over 50 years old

• 38 grams for men, or 30 grams if over 50

Recently, however, fiber has popped up in headlines thanks to people like journalist Megyn Kelly and model Molly Sims, who have both credited their physiques on mainlining roughage. And more importantly, new research has been shedding more light on how fiber helps our bodies. This nutrient has been linked to fending off disease and reducing the risk of a range of conditions, including type 2 diabetes, food allergies, and even knee arthritis.

Star-studded endorsements aside, it's not about eating a "high-fiber" diet as much as it's simply this: Eat more fiber. Fiber does more than contributing to weight loss and reducing the risk of disease.

Losing out on those recommended fiber grams per day may significantly change the way your gut functions. It could even make a difference between weight loss or none, and longer life or not.

What we know about fiber today

Many studies have strongly linked high-fiber diets with longer and healthier lives. For example, Dr. Burkitt, as mentioned above, found in the 1960s that Ugandans who ate high-fiber vegetable diets avoided many of the common diseases of Europeans and Americans. In addition, studies in the late '80s found that long-living rural Japanese populations ate high-fiber diets, as opposed to urban dwellers with lower fiber intakes.

But only recently have we gained a deeper understanding of why fiber is so vital to our well-being.

A 2017 study found that the importance of fiber is intimately tied with the importance of our gut microbes. A proper fiber diet literally feeds and makes these bacteria thrive. In turn, they increase in number and kind. The more microbes we have in our intestines, the thicker the mucus wall and the better the barrier between our body and our busy bacteria population. While the mucus barrier lowers inflammation throughout the body, the bacteria aid in digestion, creating a dual benefit.

A living, walking example of the great connection between fiber, intestinal bacteria, and health are the Hazda, a Tanzanian tribe that's one of the last remaining hunter-gatherer communities in the world. They eat a spectacular 100 grams of fiber a day, all from food sources that are seasonally available. As a result, their gut biome is packed with diverse populations of bacteria, which ebb and flow with the changing of the seasons and the changes in their diet.

Your biome can change by the season, by the week, or even by the meal. And if you eat a large array of fresh fruits, grains, and vegetables, your gut health will reflect that. Eating low-fiber foods, or eating only a few types of fiber — such as the same fiber supplement every day — can harm your intestinal biome and the health of your protective mucus wall.

However, eating too much fiber can cause digestive distress, gas, and intestinal blockages. The good news is that it's hard to get too much fiber, especially since most people don't get enough. Slowly ramping up your fiber intake can help you avoid some of the above problems. Not overdoing it will help you avoid the rest.

How to eat fiber like they do in Yuzurihara and Tanzania

So how can we ditch our constipated ways and eat more in line with how our bodies have evolved to function alongside our gut biomes? While there are two types of fiber — soluble fiber and insoluble fiber — high-fiber enthusiasts are all about both types. Each kind has its own functions and benefits. Getting both is key to getting the most out of this nutrient.

Here are some quick tips to build a thriving and diverse gut biome and reap the long-term benefits of a fiber-friendly diet:

Fruits and vegetables are always your friend

Fiber is naturally found in all fruits and vegetables. You can't really go wrong by adding these components to your daily regime. In fact, one study found that simply eating an apple before every meal had significant health benefits.

Eat what's in season

The Hazda have a diverse gut in part by eating seasonally. Always check out your grocery store's fresh, in-season fruits and veggies. Not only are they great for you, but they also often taste better and are less expensive than what's out of season.

Processed foods usually mean less fiber

Refined foods that don't contain whole grains or whole wheat are also lower in fiber. This includes white bread and regular pasta. Juicing is also processed in a sense, since it removes the insoluble fiber from your food. The result is that you lose fiber's benefits — especially its important job of regulating digestion and keeping blood sugar from spiking.

Be thoughtful at restaurants

Restaurants, especially fast-food joints, often skimp on fruits and veggies because they're expensive. When looking at the menu, be sure to pick something rich in fruit, veggies, and beans or legumes that will help you meet your fiber goals for the day.

Toss a high-fiber component into your meal

Next time you have a piece of pizza, make sure to munch on a handful of snap peas on the side, or add some multigrain crackers if you're eating soup for lunch. Eating a high-fiber snack before your meal can also mean eating fewer calories altogether, because you'll feel fuller.

Don't forget beans, peas, and lentils

We often remember to eat our fruits and veggies, but legumes are a wonderful and delicious source of fiber. Try a recipe that puts legumes in the spotlight, like a three-bean vegetarian chili or a lentil salad.

Make sure fiber starts at breakfast

Most traditional breakfast foods, like eggs and bacon, lack fiber. Integrate fiber into the first meal of your day by eating oatmeal or a whole-grain cereal. You can also simply add a piece of fruit to your regular fare. Eating yogurt for breakfast? Add sliced fruit and nuts.

Explore the world of whole grains

Next time you're at the grocery store, pick up some amaranth, bulgur, pearl barley, or wheat berries and start exploring. Other good high-fiber choices are quinoa (a seed) or whole-wheat couscous (a pasta).

Skip the fiber supplements

Fiber supplements can give you a small boost, but the benefits of getting your fiber from whole foods are much greater. What's more, people taking fiber supplements might not be pairing them with high-nutrient foods. This causes rather than solves health issues.

Too much of a good thing

Just like most things, fiber isn't great in extremely high quantities. Focusing too much on one aspect of your nutrient intake is neither sustainable nor healthy, either. Try tracking your fiber intake for a few weeks to see if you're getting enough, then tinker with your intake to see if eating a little more improves how you feel.

Fiber is fabulous without the fad

At this point, there's enough science out there to strongly suggest something you've likely heard before: Eating a robust variety of minimally processed fruits and veggies along with other plant-based foods is a great way to stay healthy and control your weight — and the fiber in these foods is likely a central reason why they're so great for our bodies. So, go forth and repopulate more varieties of bacteria in your gut!

FIBER FUELED RECIPES

Maple Granola with Banana Whipped Topping

Ingredients;

- 2 cups of rolled oats

- ¼ cup of raw sunflower seeds

- ¼ cup of raw pumpkin seeds

- ¼ cup of raw unsweetened shredded dried coconut

- ¼ cup chopped walnuts

- ¼ cup raw or toasted wheat germ

- 1 teaspoon ground cinnamon

- ½ cup maple syrup

- ¾ cup raisins

- Banana Whipped Topping, optional

For Banana Whipped Topping

- 8 ounces soft or firm regular tofu, drained (sprouted variety is preferred)

- 1 ripe banana

- 2 tablespoons maple syrup, plus more as needed

Instructions

i. Line a baking sheet with parchment paper and preheat your oven to 330 degrees F.

ii. Combine oats, pumpkin seeds, walnuts, sunflower seeds, cinnamon and wheat germ in a bowl along with maple syrup.

iii. Now in your baking sheet, spread the mixture evenly and bake for about 20 minutes.

iv. Stir in raisins and bake for another 5 minutes until the oats are golden.

v. Transfer to another baking sheet or tray and let it cool. You can serve it with banana toppings.

For Topping

Combine topping ingredients in a blender until smooth. Add maple syrup as desired

Chickpea Flour Scramble

Ingredients

Chickpea flour batter:

• ½ cup of chickpea flour or use ½ cup + 1 or 2 tablespoons of more gram flour

• ½ cup of water

• 1 tablespoon of nutritional yeast

• 1 tablespoon of flaxseed meal

• ½ teaspoon of baking powder

• ¼ teaspoon of salt

• ¼ teaspoon of turmeric

• ¼ teaspoon or less paprika

• 1/8 teaspoon of Indian Sulphur black salt for the eggy flavor

• Generous dash of black pepper

For Veggies:

• 1 teaspoon of oil divided

• 1 clove of garlic

• ¼ cup chopped onions

• 2 tablespoons each of asparagus green bell pepper, zucchini or other veggies.

• ½ green chili, chopped

• 2 tablespoons of chopped red bell pepper or tomato

• Cilantro and black pepper for garnish

Instructions

i. Blend all the ingredients under chickpea flour batter and keep aside. You can also use lentil batter from my lentil frittata.

ii. Heat ½ teaspoon of oil in a skillet over medium heat. Add onion and garlic and cook for about 3 minutes until translucent.

iii. Add veggies, chili and cook for another 2 mins, then add spices and greens.

iv. Cover the veggies with the chickpea flour batter and continue cooking while adding olive oil.

v. Since the mixture tends to get doughy, be sure to scrap the bottom. Cook until the edges dry out. This should take about 5 minutes.

vi. Turn off the stove and break the food into smaller chunks then season with salt and pepper. You can garnish with cilantro if you like. Serve with toast or tacos.

Peanut Butter and Jam Porridge

Ingredients

Peanut butter granola;

• ½ cup of rolled oats or an assortment of cereals/nuts/seeds in your pantry

• 1 tablespoon peanut butter

• 1 teaspoon of rice malt syrup

Raspberry chia jam

• ¼ cup raspberries

• 1 tablespoon chia seeds

Porridge

• ⅔ Cupof rolled oats

- 1½ cup of coconut milk

- 2 tablespoons of peanut butter (optional)

- 1 banana, mashed (optional)

Other toppings

- 2 tablespoons of peanut butter

- Whatever you desire! (Such as cacao nibs, coconut syrup, coconut and frozen berries)

Instructions

i. Preheat oven to 360°F.

ii. Combine granola ingredients in a baking sheet and bake for about 10 minutes (or until golden brown)

iii. Mash raspberries and mix in chia seeds then set it aside.

iv. Combine all porridge ingredients in a saucepan and bring to boil. Stir occasionally to maintain its smoothness.

v. Separate the porridge into 2 bowls and add granola, chia seeds, and peanut butter as desired.

Banana Almond Granola

Ingredients

- 8 cups rolled oats

- 2 cups pitted and chopped dates

- 2 ripe bananas, peeled and chopped

- 1 teaspoon almond extract

- 1 teaspoon salt

- 1 cup slivered almonds, toasted (optional)

Instructions

i. Preheat the oven to 275°F.

ii. Line a baking sheet with parchment paper.

iii. Cook dates covered with water in a saucepan over medium heat for about 10 minutes. Make sure the dates do not stick on the pan.

iv. Take the mixture off heat and in a blender, combine it with almond extract, bananas and salt until creamy.

v. Add oats to the date mixture and spread out on the baking sheet. Bake for about 45 minutes – occasionally stirring.

vi. Remove from oven and let it cool. Enjoy.

Polenta with Pears and Cranberries

Ingredients

- ¼ cup of brown rice syrup

- 2 pears, peeled, cored, and diced

- 1 cup of fresh or dried cranberries

- 1 teaspoon ground cinnamon

- 1 batch Basic Polenta, kept warm

Instructions

i. In a medium saucepan, combine the brown rice syrup, cranberries, pears and cinnamon. Cook until the pears are tender.

ii. Divide as desired and top with pear compote.

Fruit and Nut Oatmeal

Ingredients

- ¾ cup of rolled oats

- ¼ teaspoon ground cinnamon

- Pinch of sea salt

- ¼ cup fresh berries (optional)

- ½ ripe banana, sliced (optional)

- 2 tablespoons of chopped nuts, such as walnuts, pecans, or cashews (optional)

- 2 tablespoons of dried fruit, such as raisins, cranberries, chopped apples, chopped

- Apricots (optional)

- Maple syrup (optional)

Instructions

i. Cook oats in water in a saucepan until it starts boiling. Reduce the heat and let it simmer for about 5 minutes.

ii. Add cinnamon and salt – stirring. Top with berries and fruits and serve while hot.

Red Pesto and Kale Porridge

Ingredients

- ½ cup of oats
- ½ cup of couscous
- 2 cups of veggie stock (or water)
- 1 teaspoon of dried oregano
- 1 teaspoon of dried basil
- 1 cup of chopped kale
- 1 cup of sliced cherry tomatoes
- 1 scallion
- 1 teaspoon of tahini
- 1 tablespoon of pesto of your choice

* 2 tablespoons of nutritional yeast

* 1 tablespoon of pumpkin seed

* 1 tablespoon of hemp seed

* Salt and pepper to taste

Instructions

i. Cook oats, couscous, vegetable stock, oregano, basil, salt and pepper in a small pot on medium heat for about 5 minutes stirring occasionally.

ii. Once it becomes creamy, add scallions, chopped kale, and tomatoes. Stir in pesto, yeast, and tahini.

iii. Top with some cherry tomatoes hemp seeds and pumpkin and serve it warm.

Spicy Tofu Scramble

Ingredients

* 350g of firm tofu

* 2 small spring onions, sliced

- 1 large garlic clove, finely chopped

- 10 cherry tomatoes, halved

- ½ fresh red chili, sliced

- 1 avocado, sliced

- 1 teaspoon of ground turmeric

- 2 teaspoon of ground black salt

- Salt & pepper to taste

- 1 to 2 tablespoons of olive oil

- 8 slices of gluten-free bread, toasted

Instructions

i. Sauté garlic in olive oil in a pan.

ii. Add in tomatoes and cook until they're soft then remove the mixture from the pan.

iii. Under a grill, toast bread slices. Sauté some onions and chili seeds on low-medium heat until they soften and add tofu.

iv. Sprinkle with turmeric and black salt and stir it for a couple of minutes. Finally, add tomatoes and garlic back to the pan to warm up.

v. Add the tofu scramble onto the toasted bread slices and decorate with avocado. Season as desired. Enjoy!

Green Chia Pudding

Ingredients

• 1 Medjool date with pit removed

• 1 cup non-dairy milk organic soy, almond, or coconut

• 1 handful fresh spinach

• 3 tablespoons of chia seeds

• Fruit for topping banana, kiwi, mango or berries

Instructions

i. Combine the dates, milk, and spinach in a blender until smooth then add it to chia seeds in a medium bowl.

ii. Store in the refrigerator for up to overnight.

iii. Top with fruit before serving.

Turmeric Steel Cut Oats

Ingredients

• ¼ teaspoon of olive oil

• ½ cup of steel cut oats use certified gluten-free if needed

• 1½ cup of water 2 cups for a thinner consistency

• 1 cup of non-dairy milk

• 1/3 teaspoon of turmeric

• ½ teaspoon of cinnamon

• ¼ teaspoon of cardamom

• Salt to taste

• 2 tablespoons or more, of maple or other sweetener of your choice

Instructions

i. Toast oats in oil in a saucepan for a couple of minutes.

ii. Add water and milk and bring it to a boil before letting it simmer.

iii. Mix in the spices, salt, and maple and cook for about 8 minutes or until the oats are cooked to preference.

iv. Taste and adjust sweet, and flavors as desired then let it cool to thicken. You can serve warm or chilled.

v. Garnish with strawberries, dried fruit or chia seeds

Mashed Cauliflower and Green Bean Casserole

Ingredients

- ¾ cup of coconut milk

- ½ cup of nutritional yeast

- 1 cauliflower

- Salt and pepper to taste

- 14 ounces of green beans, trimmed

- 1 onion, diced

Instructions

i. In a skillet, cook cauliflower florets in vegetable broth and some olive oil.

ii. Add in onions and beans and cook for a little longer. Transfer the mixture into a blender and add coconut milk, nutritional yeast, salt and pepper and blend until smooth.

Iii. In a baking sheet, assemble green bean mix, mashed cauliflower, and toppings and bake for 15 to 20 minutes at 400 degrees F. Enjoy.

Zucchini Noodles with Portobello Bolognese

Ingredients

• 3 tablespoons extra virgin olive oil, divided

• 6 Portobello mushroom caps, stems, and gills removed and finely chopped

• ½ cup of minced carrot

• ½ cup of minced celery

• ½ cup of minced yellow onion

- 3 large garlic cloves, minced

- Kosher salt

- Fresh ground pepper

- 1 tablespoon of tomato paste

- A 28-ounce can-crushed tomatoes (I strongly recommend San Marzano)

- 2 teaspoons of dried oregano

- ¼ teaspoon of crushed red pepper (optional)

- ½ cup fresh basil leaves, finely chopped (plus extra for serving)

- 4 medium zucchini

Instructions

i. Sauté garlic, mushrooms, celery, and carrots in olive oil in a pan. Season with salt and pepper as desired. Continue cooking until vegetables are soft.

ii. Stir in some tomato paste and cook for a couple of minutes before adding crushed tomatoes, oregano, red pepper, and basil.

iii. Let it simmer for 10 to 15 minutes until the sauce thickens.

iv. As the sauce simmers, use an appropriate blade to make spiral zucchini.

v. Sauté the zucchini noodles in a separate saucepan for a couple of minutes and season as desired.

vi. Top with a generous amount of Bolognese and garnish with freshly chopped basil and serve immediately

Burrito Bowl

Ingredients

- Baked tortilla chips

- 2 to 4 cups cooked grains

- 2 to 4 cups cooked beans

- 2 to 4 cups chopped romaine lettuce or steamed kale

- 2 to 4 chopped tomatoes

- 1 to 2 chopped green onions

- 1 to 2 cups corn kernels

- 1 avocado, chopped

- Fresh salsa

Instructions

i. Break some tortilla chips and place in a bowl.

ii. Add some cooked grains and beans.

iii. Layer on tomatoes, lettuce, corn, onions, avocado and then top with salsa.

Thai Noodles

Ingredients

- 8 ounces brown rice noodles or other whole-grain noodles

- 3 tablespoons of low-sodium soy sauce, or to taste

- 2 tablespoons of brown rice syrup or maple syrup

- 2 tablespoons of fresh lime juice (from 1 to 2 limes)

- 4 garlic cloves, minced

- 3 cups of frozen Asian-style vegetables

- 1 cup of mung bean sprouts

- 2 green onions, white and light green parts chopped

- 3 tablespoons of chopped, roasted, unsalted peanuts

- ¼ cup of chopped fresh cilantro

- 1 lime, cut into wedges

Instructions

i. Follow instructions for cooking noodles.

ii. Combine soy sauce, garlic, brown rice syrup, lime juice and cup water and bring to a boil. Stir in the veggies and cook for about 5 minutes or until crisp-tender.

iii. Add the cooked noodles and mung bean sprouts and toss to coat then let it cook for a couple more minutes.

iv. Garnish with cilantro, green onions, lime wedges and chopped peanuts.

Mediterranean Vegetable Spaghetti

Ingredients

- 10 ounces brown rice spaghetti

- 1 red bell pepper, cubed small

- 1 yellow bell pepper, cubed small

- 2 plum tomatoes, sliced into eighths (discard the seeds)

- Salt

- ½ jalapeño (optional)

- 2 tablespoons of dried herbs de Provence

- 2 tablespoons of tomato purée

- 2 tablespoons apple cider vinegar or juice of 1 lime

- 12 cherry tomatoes, quartered

- 1 zucchini, halved then sliced into thin half-rounds

- 1 bunch spinach, chopped

- Handful of black olives

Instructions

i. Cook pasta, drain and set aside.

ii. Sauté peppers, tomatoes, jalapeno, and herbs in a saucepan. Add water and let it simmer.

iii. Add tomato puree and vinegar or lime juice and let it cook together for a few minutes until it becomes saucy.

iv. Add cherry tomatoes, zucchini slices, and spinach. Mix well and cook for about 5 to 7 minutes.

v. Add olives and sauce to the pasts along with some herbs. Enjoy

Mexican Lentil Soup

Ingredients

- 2 tablespoons extra virgin olive oil

- 1 yellow onion, diced

- 2 carrots, peeled and diced

- 2 celery stalks, diced

- 1 red bell pepper, diced

- 3 cloves garlic, minced

- 1 tablespoon cumin

- ¼ teaspoon smoked paprika

- 1 teaspoon oregano

- 2 cups diced tomatoes and the juices

- 4 ounces diced green chilies

- 2 cups green lentils, rinsed and picked over

- 8 cups vegetable broth

- ½ teaspoon salt

- A dash (or more) of hot sauce, plus more for serving

- Fresh cilantro, for garnish

- 1 avocado, peeled, pitted, and diced, or garnish

Instructions

i. Sauté onions, celery, bell pepper and carrots in a pan for about 5 minutes then add garlic, cumin, paprika, and oregano and let it cook for another minute.

ii. Add in tomatoes, chilies, lentils, broth, and salt to taste and bring to a simmer until lentils are tender.

iii. Season with salt and pepper as necessary

iv. Serve it garnished with fresh cilantro, avocado, and a few dashes of hot sauce.

CONCLUSION

When you think of the F word, it's time to start thinking about fiber. Dr. B offers us the science behind why fiber and gut health are both the way towards a healthier lifestyle, but he also gives us a solid plan to follow to reach optimum health.

And yes, transitioning to a plant-based diet may admittedly be challenging to start. There may also be some unwanted side effects, associated with upping beans and cruciferous veggies, such as gas and bloating. Dr. B's advice is to start low and go slow. Begin the process by slowly adding small quantities of fiber to your diet, so the gut can adapt to processing this efficiently.

Dr. B argues that we're only as healthy as our guts, and often we neglect just how important they're to overall health and wellness. To support the gut, we need to look after our microbes. We also need to be aware of the adverse effects that medication and poor diet can cause. Although it may seem prescriptive, following a plant-based diet is all about variety. So, embrace diversity, consume a high-fiber plant-based diet that includes an abundance of vegetables, fruit, nuts, seeds, and whole grains.